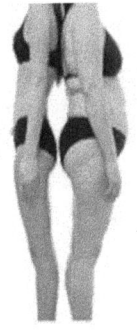

The Belly Fat, Stress And Adrenal Fatigue Solution

BY Ross Craft

About The Author

The author, Ross Craft is the survivor of blindness and two usually terminal diseases. The autoimmune disease he was diagnosed with was controlled with medications that suppress the immune system.

The medically induced enhanced adrenal function resulted in classic symptoms of adrenal fatigue as a side effect of the drugs. The most obvious effect was massive weight gain around the belly and a fat face or moon face.

Once he recovered, and stopped the medications he still had to deal with the excess belly fat caused by the prolonged elevated cortisol levels. His research led him to Dr. James Wilsons and the explanation of adrenal fatigue.

Please refer to his blog at http://binauralbeats.mobi for information and binaural beats recordings.

Please refer to
http://www.learningtodanceintherain.com for more on his inspiring story.

Table of Contents

Introduction

Do any of these sound familiar to you?

Weight gain, especially around the middle section, with extreme difficulty in losing it
Morning fatigue – not seeming to wake up until 10:00AM even though you have been up three hours
Middle of the afternoon LUL
Sluggishness, cloudy thinking in the middle of the day
Burst of energy around 6PM
Sleepiness around 9PM but a second burst of energy about 11pm to 1am. You may find it difficult to fall asleep between those times.
Mild depression
Decreased sex drive, lack of energy and lack of focus and concentration
Muscular weakness and declining endurance
Unrelaxing and unfulfilling sleep.

While I am sure some of us can relate to a few of these, it is scary to think how many people suffer from three or more of these warning signs. Even worse is that some of you can relate to all of these.

For many of us, the most obvious sign of adrenal fatigue is excess fat around the belly.

Dr. James L. Wilson coined the term "ADRENAL FATIGUE" in 1998 to identify a group of signs and symptoms that people experience as a result of decreased adrenal function. This lack of adrenal performance is often associated with the affects of stress on the human body.

Adrenal fatigue can affect anyone who experiences frequent, persistent or severe mental, emotional or physical stress. It can also be an important contributing factor in health conditions ranging from allergies to undesirable weight gain with increased belly fat. Despite its prevalence in our modern world, adrenal fatigue has generally been ignored and misunderstood by the medical community. In order to help the many individuals experiencing the problem, this ebook was written to raise awareness of "This 21st Century Syndrome" and to recommend a very simple easy solution.

You may not be able to change your lifestyle to relieve your stress but you can easily increase your capacity to handle stress.

Chapter 1 –Stress Creeps In

If you are like most Americans you can probably remember your youth as a carefree time, you had little responsibility and the biggest concern was the date plan for Saturday night.

As these days faded into the distant memory many Americans find themselves caught in a seemingly endless race.

The mornings are usually a marathon of routines and rituals. Hitting the snooze button for an extra 20 minutes of sleep, rushing through errands hoping to get out of the house a few minutes early and grabbing a quick cup of coffee and breakfast sandwich at a fast food restaurant. Only on rare days do you make it out early enough to beat the congestion and traffic and accidents that seem to be at a growing rate of road rage.

Once you get to work, you throw yourself into a gauntlet of endless tasks and projects and stringent deadlines to maintain some semblance of job security. You then take a quick lunch break, taking just the minimum amount of time state laws require – just enough time to down a sandwich and a soda or two.

By the end of the day you are exhausted and left to face the same nightmare on roads that stressed you that morning. You then might retreat to your home reassuring yourself that tonight will be different. Tonight you will have the time to relax and enjoy your downtime, but you come home only to see the bills piling up on the counter. You have to address the problem your child had at school, your spouse is also stressed and ready to snap.

By the time you have taken care of everything you might be able to watch a few minutes of late night television as you unwind and try to force yourself to get to sleep at a decent hour.

One of the most significant problems most Americans face each day is the battery of stress that attacks us from almost every angle. While you may think that you are personally strong and able to face stressors without any problems, your body might not agree.

In the past century, science and private industry has turned out an almost infinite number of inventions, tools, electronics and even drugs each designed to improve our lifestyles, all they seem to do is make life more fast paced.

The problem with today's lifestyle is there are millions of products and businesses that provide convenience, but with each convenience comes a significant cost. Fast food is fast and cheap and available in minutes, but the nutrients are severely lacking and it is loaded with saturated fat, sugar and excessive calories.

Computers continue to become faster and smarter than most of us need, but rather than allowing us to work more leisurely, we are expected to perform more work in the same amount of time or multitask (do two things at once).
While our tools, equipment and food become faster and smarter the basic chemistry of our bodies remains the same.

We can always work longer, harder and even smarter, but the human body was not designed to handle this, at least to the degree that society often demands.

With a barrage of stress, lack of exercise, unbalanced diet and a day to day lifestyle that leaves little time to relax, your body may be ready to call it quits.

Most of us get a week or two of vacation time per year, hoping that this little time will be enough time to unwind and recharge. Does this sound like you? If so, your body may be in trouble.

Chapter – 2 – The Adrenal System

One of the most overlooked and overworked systems in the body is the adrenal system. This may sound familiar because you may have heard of adrenalin which is exclusively controlled by the adrenal glands, but how much do you really know about your adrenal system.

While adrenalin is mainly utilized as the primary energy source in an emergency, there is that rush of excitement, fast heart rate and surge of energy you get before a close call that almost resulted in a traffic accident, or when a housewife is able to lift the front of a car as it pins her child to the ground.

The adrenal glands are also solely responsible for the production and management of Cortisol, which is the body's primary defense system to help fight stress.

In addition, the adrenal glands greatly influence the body's ability to maintain steady energy throughout the day. Most of us overstress our adrenal glands everyday thru poor diet, intake of caffeine and other stimulants, stress, lack of sleep and other energy robbing activities. Think about it, when was the last time you took a minute to refresh this overtaxed system.

Generally speaking, as the adrenal system continues to be overtaxed it is unable to keep up with production. Like a production line that is severely understaffed, the adrenal glands can only function so long above their means until production suffers.

When the adrenal system is unable to function completely it is unable to manage the energy your lifestyle is demanding. As the adrenal glands fatigue the production of response hormones decline.

The most significant causes of adrenal fatigue are constant physical or emotional stress, the overuse of stimulants and nicotine, lack of exercise and a poor diet.

For most people adrenal fatigue is caused by a combination of these factors. However everyone responds to each of these stressors differently. It is even possible to reach this stage with zero caffeine and stimulant intake. With the right combination of physical and emotional stressors, lack of sleep and poor lifestyle, it is just as easy to burn out your adrenal glands while stimulant free.

Some people feel little effect from physical and emotional stress, yet their lack of exercise poor diet and stimulant abuse are key contributors in damaging their adrenal glands.

It is important to realize that you might think that you handle stress well, but truly it takes a major toll on the body. There are not always clear cut signs that the body is facing stress. As the adrenal glands fatigue you may also notice some signs of depression as your energy decreases, you might have trouble staying motivated, your outlook on life is somewhat grim, you become irritable over miner things, you have a disinterest in hobbies and pleasurable activities including sex.

Besides symptoms of depression, you are probably noticing increased weight gain, especially around your middle and you are finding it hard to shed this fat.

Why is this all happening? Is this just the normal signs of aging?
The answer is NO!

In the next chapters we will cover how your adrenal system serves almost like the bodies control center, how with binaural beats meditation you can increase your stress tolerance capacity, greatly improve your energy levels and make you feel young and vibrant.

Chapter -3- The Endocrine System and the Adrenal Glands

The endocrine system is a system of glands throughout your body responsible for the release of hormones. As a whole the endocrine system is responsible for regulating metabolism, energy production and even significant in many aspects of controlling your mood.

The adrenal system is an important part of the endocrine system. So, what is the adrenal system? Where are your adrenal glands? When asked, many people point to their neck, possibly confusing their adrenal glands with their thyroid, but your adrenal glands are located in your abdomen right above your kidneys.

A normal functioning adrenal is irresponsible for the release of dopamine. Dopamine in the brain has been shown to play an important role in cognition, motor function, motivation, sleep, mood, attention and learning. If your adrenal function is repressed and your dopamine levels are lower than normal, you may experience symptoms of depression, fatigue and lack of motivation.

Proper dopamine levels are one of the key components in maintaining a positive outlook on life. The hormones secreted by the adrenalin system control the body's response to stress including the fight or flight adrenalin surge when you face danger or stress.

The outer part of the adrenal gland is the adrenal cortex, which produces a number of different hormones, such as, Cortisol, aldostrane and DHEA. These hormones carefully control metabolism and other characteristics, such as, hair growth and body shape. DHEA is often called the mother hormone since it has the ability to convert into sex hormones, such as, testosterone and estrogen as needed.

Studies have shown that DHEA is increased with regular exercise and the average adult produces about 25mg a day. Adequate levels of DHEA are needed to assure your body can produce the proper hormones it needs to function properly.

When the body's hormones are balanced your mood is constant and you feel lucid, constant and enthusiastic. DHEA is considered by many to be the best feel good hormone in the body. When DHEA levels are low due to improper adrenal function your body cannot regulate proper body function. Improper hormone function can cause you to experience a sense of depression and melancholy.

One of the main hormones produced by the adrenal system is Cortisol. While Cortisol is an essential hormone, if its levels are not balanced in the body it can cause serious health concerns.

Cortisol is the primary stress hormone. Its primary function is to restore stability or homeostasis after stress. To accomplish this task, Cortisol raises blood pressure, increases blood sugar, weakens the immune system, slows the metabolism and even impairs memory and thinking.

While these are all negative effects, in an emergency these drastic changes help the body eliminate escape or cope with stress. Cortisol is essential for survival, but chronically elevated Cortisol levels can seriously injure your health.

When you are stressed your body releases Cortisol to control the stress response. But, what happens when you are constantly stressed? Cortisol levels remain elevated. Looking at Cortisol's function you can see why elevated levels of this hormone are very bad for your health.

Not only will it cause you to gain weight, it hinders your metabolism and can even weaken your immune system. This formula makes you susceptible to illness, while making it almost impossible to control your weight.

While Cortisol can damage the body it is necessary in its intended dose. Cortisol is essential for controlling blood sugar levels because of its ability to control insulin. Serving as the primary hormone in response to stress our bodies need Cortisol to survive emergencies.

In the past some products have attempted to cure stress induced weight gain by blocking or eliminating Cortisol. Without Cortisol your insulin levels would remain elevated for hours after eating and insulin signals the body to pack food (glucose) into the cells. This will again just lead to weight gain.

Rather than eliminate Cortisol the healthy way to control weight, energy, mood and sleep is to allow Cortisol to function in the body within the normal realm if its function. We want Cortisol, just not too much or too little.

Chapter -4- Factors Affecting The Adrenal Glands.

There are several lifestyle factors that can significantly influence or modify adrenal function. When continued stress increases the normal function of the adrenal glands it forces the glands to produce more output, produce more energy and increase the output of stress and response hormones. With minor stress reactions this is a normal process, as it is what the adrenal glands were designed to do.

When you give your body adequate time to recover the adrenal glands revert back to normal functioning, as well as, normal energy production.

When the adrenal glands are not given the time and tools necessary to recover they may weaken over time. Then their functionality may become exhausted.

By definition, all stimulants like, caffeine and nicotine are drugs that have the ability to increase the activity of the central nervous system and /or the sympathetic nervous system. For instance, let's look at a stimulant everyone is familiar with, caffeine. Caffeine is a natural substance as it is found in over 60 plants. The caffeine that you and I most commonly consume is extracted from the beans of the coffee plant and/or the leaves of tea bushes.

When you consume caffeine it is absorbed in the stomach and small intestines. It usually takes 15 minutes for caffeine to produce its stimulating effect. Just how long does that caffeine stay in your system? On average, the half life of caffeine is between 3 and 4 hours in a healthy adult. However, this number nearly doubles to 5 to 10 hours in women taking oral contraceptives. What this means is every 3 to 4 hours 50% of the caffeine is being eliminated.

After consuming 100mg of caffeine, the average cup of coffee, it can take up to 15 hours before the caffeine is completely metabolized. The higher dose you consume the longer the process will take.

So when you have a soda or cup of coffee in the afternoon, there are still stimulants in your system when you go to bed in the evening.

You can see how stimulants earlier in the day can contribute to sleep disorders.

There is no question that caffeine and other stimulants have some very attractive benefits to us. They allow us to work faster, be more alert, typically raise our mood, alleviate headaches, and reduce our awareness of stress, but with most benefits come a compromise. Stimulants such as caffeine can play a significant role in your body's adenosine management. Adenosine is your bodies control center. Adenosine plays a major role producing deep restful sleep and suppressing the body's tendency to get restless sleep.

When adenosine is not received properly in the body energy levels decrease and sleep quality can decrease. The effects of adenosine have been shown to be significantly blunted in individuals who were taking large quantities of stimulants like caffeine, green tea, nicotine and amphetamines.

Chapter -5- Life style contributions

Stimulants are not the only things that have an effect on adrenal health. While stimulants can be the easiest target, an equal if not greater amount of damage can be contributed to your lifestyle.

As we covered, the adrenal glands are responsible for the fight or flight response that is one of the most important tools in survival. The fight or flight response is the triggered response you get when you stand in certain danger. Chemical reactions take place in milliseconds and the body quickly reacts to the danger at hand.

When the body is stressed and the fight or flight response is triggered the body responds quickly. Heart rate increases, arteries and veins allow maximum blood flow, breathing rate increases bringing more oxygen to the lungs and muscles faster, fat and sugars are metabolized to create instant energy, pupils dilate to give better vision, the digestive system is slowed to provide energy , sweat glands are activated, endorphins are released, mental judgment and clarity is delayed. This is very interesting because the body reacts to daily stressors in a similar way.

When the body is mentally and emotionally stressed, it releases hormones to try to combat the situation and maintain homeostasis or a stable functioning condition that is normal until one of two things happen. The body exhausts or the stress is relieved.

Sleep is one of the most important aspects of our lives, yet we seem to give it the least amount of attention. Most of us sleep on twelve year old mattresses, flat pillows and get far too little sleep per night. The notion of catching up on the weekends is almost as farfetched as putting this book under your pillow and expecting it will be committed to memory by morning.

Sleep is the only true resting period your body gets. It is the body's only time to repair, grow and relax. Think about how much brain activity it takes just to read this sentence. Muscles in your eyes scan the page, pupils adjust to the light in the room, the retina transmits the characters to a series of nerves which transmit the findings to the brain. Your brain recognizes the characters, translates their meaning and creates ideas and emotions based upon the text.

Simultaneously your hands are holding the book, other muscles are holding your posture up so you can sit without keeling over, your breathing is steady and your blood is pumping thru miles of arteries, veins and capillaries. At the same time your brain is aware of the temperature in the room, the texture of your clothes, and the comfort of your chair or background noises. Your brain is constantly working all day long. Even when you are doing the most mundane tasks, there are millions of processes going on each second.

Once you consider the abuse your brain goes thru all day long just for you to function smoothly, don't you think sleep is the least you can do for it?

Consider the intensified impact that stimulants and stress play on your body each day. The human body was engineered to reset during the hours of sleep. Some people need 8 hours of sleep each night and others operate great on lonely 6. We do accept that everyone is similar at their core. Yet, we must identify the fact that every person is different.

While the duration of the number of hours you sleep is extremely important, the most important factor of sleep is the quality of sleep.

So, as you continue to live and push yourself at a greater pace just to keep up, your body continues to work harder and harder to provide the energy and mental ingenuity for you to succeed. Most of us take for granted the endurance our adrenal glands provide for us daily. Yet after a barrage of stimulants from coffee, sodas and diet pills running a gauntlet of projects and tasks at work without taking adequate time to relax and a home life that is typically far from relaxing, at this point your adrenal glands may be exhausted.

Chapter 6 - The Solution – Binaural Beats Meditation!!

Most of us are living a 21st century life pace with 19th century coping skills. To resolve this problem, it is not necessary to get out of the "race", but it is necessary to learn how to live with the ever increasing pace of life that produces stress for most of us.

Luckily, you can increase your stress tolerance quickly and easily. It is well documented that meditation is one of the most powerful antidotes to stress. And binaural beats meditation is even more powerful in this regard than traditional meditation.

Meditation methods like yoga and transcendental meditation are effective but generally require a learning curve or years of practice to get the most benefit. On the other hand, scientists have discovered that listening to the proper sound at the proper frequency will naturally guide or entrain our brains to relax into the same meditative state as those achieved by long time meditators. The best part is, you can think about anything you want during this process. In addition, you don't have to understand or believe anything, it just happens naturally. This is definitely the modern day answer to stress relief and the benefits are amazing.

It has been established that 20 minutes of deep meditation is physically and mentally equivalent to 3 hours of sleep. With binaural beats meditation you can meditate like a Zen master the very first time and every time you try.

Meditation dramatically lowers stress and stress-related physical and emotional problems, say research scientists in thousands of studies. Several studies are included below, just to give an indication of the stature of the researchers.

> The National Institute of Health reports that regular meditation can reduce chronic pain, anxiety, high blood pressure, cholesterol, health care use, substance abuse, post traumatic stress response, and blood levels of stress hormones.

> Frank Treiber, Phd., of Medical College of Georgia, says that meditation lowers blood pressure, even for healthy young people, creating a 12.5% lower risk of stroke or coronary mortality in adulthood.

Cedars-Sinai Medical Center researchers say meditation improves stress response, "similar to the physiological impact of exercise conditioning."

Researchers at the University Of Maryland School Of Medicine report that meditation relieved stress, reduced rheumatoid arthritis symptoms, reduced cardiovascular risk factors, decreased psychological distress, improved sleep patterns.

The Mayo Clinic Health Letter says that meditation reduces high blood pressure, anxiety, substance abuse, post-tramatic stress syndrome, and visits to health care providers

Dr. Herbert Benson of Harvard Medical School found that meditation releases tension, and creates the will power and consciousness to be in control of one's life and alleviates depression, loneliness, hopelessness and despair.

Ninety cancer patients who meditated for 7 weeks had 31% lower stress symptoms and 67% less mood disturbance than those who did not meditate.

Other studies have shown that meditation lowers elevated Cortisol levels

Meditation with binaural beats is based on the natural characteristics of the mind to react to sound. Since the beginning of time, man has responded to the beat of the drum. The tendency of the mind to follow and synchronize with the rhythm of beats led scientists to develop sounds that will help you relax into a desired mental state.

Further research revealed that specific parts of the brain or specific Neuro pathways could be stimulated with specific sounds. Using the frequency following response, you can meditate like a long time meditator on your first try. As you exercise the proper Neuro pathways you will raise your stress tolerance point, your happiness set point and you can even increase your IQ by as much as 25% by listening to the sound that exercises that part of your brain.

Chapter -7- Meditation – Self Growth for Busy People

Binaural beats meditation stimulates the brain but, it isn't just any stimulation. It is holistic in that it not only exercises the desired area of the brain, but it also exercises all areas the same as in traditional meditation. It's a stimulation that causes the two sides of the brain to become more synchronized, more balanced.

> This creates what scientists call "whole brain thinking", with new intelligence, perspectives, and focus and an increased ability of creative thinking, higher intelligence and spiritual awareness.

> This is why focus and concentration increase when people listen to binaural beats meditation recordings. This is why problem solving ability increases. This is why creativity and learning increase.

> It is also why positive emotions increase and negative emotions fall away.

With Meditation your brain is practicing making alpha waves, so it becomes more skilled at doing it. More alpha waves mean:

Faster learning,

Greater ability to focus,

More joy,

More happiness and

More inner peace.

You are also learning to make more theta waves when you listen to Meditation recordings,

Which means more creativity,

A greater ability to bond with others and

A greater ability to experience how you fit into the universe and

How it all goes together.

Finally, your brain is learning to make more delta waves.

This leads to deep spiritual experience.

It is also the brainwave pattern of incredible persuasiveness.

Meditation has a dramatic and positive effect on stress and the physical and emotional problems caused by stress!!

Given the ever increasing pace of life in the 21st century, we all need to become more resilient, more stress resistant. The evidence is clear: meditation is the best of all available stress-busting tools and with continued use our stress tolerance is increased. It is the indispensable 21st century coping skill.

It is easy to protect yourself from Adrenal Fatigue and get rid of that extra fat tire around your middle along with all the stress-related physical and mental problems associated with the ever increasing pace of life. You will find that everything just works better and that extra fat around your middle will be the first to go as your cortisol levels normalize and your whole life improves.

Chapter -8- Be All You Can Be

After the very first meditation session you can expect to feel the way you would feel when you wake up from a very nice nap.   In the short 20 to 30 minutes you will feel refreshed.

With continued meditations, you will likely notice things like the beauty of flowers; you had just been walking past without notice. Meditation practioners call this expanded awareness. You might also realize while on your morning commute you do not get an emotional response when someone cuts you off. You might just think, that guy must be late for work I hope he makes it. That is when you may realize you are getting increased stress tolerance. You might also realize you have less stress when you get home and your partner starts looking really good.

At work you may start feeling more in control of your tasks and the fast pace will not seem as fast. When you can do more work in less time without feeling rushed or overwhelmed you have less stress to take home and your whole life improves.   You laugh more, you are more at ease and you are a delightful person to be around.

This is the person you were meant to be and it is the person you will become. The secret is to get that extra rest that relieves all the daily stress the same day it happens. It is the accumulative effect of elevated stress levels that affect our lives and our health.

With increased will power, the next time you start a diet staying on it will be easy. The same diet that didn't seem to work before, will work like a charm.

You can become the person you know deep down you were meant to be.

The end